Shrink That Sucker (Without Shrinking Your Fun!)

A Guide to Embracing Your Socks-with-Sandals-Wearing, Karaoke-Singing Self for Better Mental Health (and Possibly World Domination) (American Edition)

Volodymyr Rybaiev

Table of Contents

Introduction: Buns of Steel...Maybe Later: Shedding Pounds Without Shedding Tears (and Your Sanity)

Let's face it, folks, the whole weight loss thing can feel like a never-ending uphill battle. You're bombarded with fad diets promising lightning-fast results, gym memberships that bleed your wallet dry, and enough confusing fitness jargon to make your head spin. It's enough to send anyone running for the donut shop (or maybe that's just me?).

But what if I told you there's a better way? A way to shrink that sucker (your waistline, that is) without shrinking your fun, your sanity, or your bank account? Buckle up, because this book is your guide to ditching the tears and the drama, and embracing a healthy lifestyle that feels, dare I say, **enjoyable**.

We'll ditch the complicated mumbo jumbo and translate all that science stuff into plain English. We'll expose the myths that have been holding you back for years (spoiler alert: kale smoothies aren't a magic bullet). And most importantly, we'll remind you that you're not alone in this journey. We'll be your partner in crime, your cheerleader, and your sassy sidekick, cracking jokes and wiping away sweat (or maybe just tears of laughter) along the way.

This book is all about progress, not perfection. We'll talk about setting realistic goals, making sustainable changes, and learning to love your body at every stage of the game. Because let's be honest, buns of steel are great and all, but a healthy dose of self-love is the real prize.

So, ditch the crash diets and the self-loathing. Let's grab a metaphorical margarita (or a glass of water, whichever you prefer) and get started on this weight loss adventure together. We're about to rewrite the rules and prove that healthy living can be fun, effective, and maybe even a little bit hilarious.

The Land of Dieting Denial: Busting Myths and Facing Facts

Farewell, Fad Diets: Why Kale Smoothies Won't Make Your Jeans Fit Like Magic

Ah, the siren song of the fad diet. It whispers sweet nothings in your ear, promising a beach bod in a blink and a wardrobe filled with clothes two sizes too small. It might involve grapefruit and cabbage soup, or maybe it's all about cutting out carbs entirely. Whatever the flavor, fad diets have one thing in common: they're about as reliable as a used car salesman with a comb-over.

Let's face it, folks, if there was a magic bullet for weight loss, wouldn't we all be strutting around in swimsuits year-round? But the reality is, there's no one-size-fits-all solution. Fad diets are like those brightly colored plastic sunglasses you bought at the beach as a kid – trendy for a hot minute, then left gathering dust in a drawer somewhere.

So, why exactly are fad diets a recipe for disaster? Let's grab a metaphorical scalpel and dissect the reasons why they'll leave you feeling frustrated and reaching for the ice cream carton faster than you can say "yo-yo effect."

The Unsustainable Charade:

Fad diets are all about extremes. They demonize entire food groups (carbs, I'm looking at you!), restrict calories to starvation levels, and promise results that sound more like science fiction than healthy living. The problem? These extremes are, well, extreme. They're almost impossible to stick with in the long run. Imagine surviving on nothing but grapefruit and tuna for weeks on end. Sounds delightful, right? (Spoiler alert: It's not.)

Most people who embark on these restrictive journeys end up feeling deprived, cranky, and ready to throw in the towel at the first sight of a birthday cake. The result? A binge-fest of epic proportions and a renewed sense of guilt. It's a vicious cycle, friends, and one you don't want to get stuck in.

The Myth of Magic Bullets:
Here's the truth bomb: there's no magic pill, potion, or smoothie
that will melt away fat overnight. Don't get me wrong, kale
smoothies can be a healthy addition to your diet, but they're not
some magical elixir that will magically transform your body.
Weight loss is a marathon, not a sprint. It requires consistent
effort, healthy habits, and a sustainable approach.
Fad diets often focus on quick fixes and ignore the underlying
causes of weight gain. They don't teach you about portion
control, mindful eating, or building a balanced diet. They don't
address factors like stress, sleep, and exercise, all of which play a
crucial role in maintaining a healthy weight.

The War on Nutrients:
Many fad diets demonize entire food groups, often based on
flawed science or trendy marketing tactics. Remember the Atkins
craze that vilified carbs? While it might have led to some initial
weight loss, it also came with potential downsides like nutrient
deficiencies, bad breath, and increased risk of kidney stones.
Our bodies need a variety of nutrients to function properly. Carbs
provide energy, protein helps build and repair tissues, and
healthy fats keep us feeling full and satisfied. Cutting out entire
food groups can leave you feeling sluggish, irritable, and craving
the very things you're trying to avoid.

The Yo-Yo Effect Blues:
Let's be honest, the rapid weight loss promised by fad diets often
comes with a not-so-fun side effect: the yo-yo effect. You restrict
your calories, lose weight quickly, then inevitably get tired of
feeling like a hangry monster. So, you ditch the diet, go back to
your old ways, and guess what? The weight comes back with a
vengeance, often bringing some unwelcome friends (hello, extra
pounds!).
This constant cycle of restriction and overindulgence can wreak
havoc on your metabolism and leave you feeling discouraged. It's
a demoralizing rollercoaster that can seriously impact your
relationship with food and your body.

The Recipe for Success:

So, what's the alternative to fad diets? The good news is, there's a whole world of healthy and sustainable weight loss strategies waiting to be explored. We're talking about making gradual changes, building healthy habits, and learning to love your body at every stage of the journey.

This book will be your guide on this adventure. We'll ditch the confusing jargon and break down the science of weight loss into plain English. We'll explore tips for portion control, smart grocery shopping, and creating a balanced diet that actually tastes good. We'll talk about the importance of exercise, but we'll also focus on finding activities you actually enjoy (because let's be real, nobody enjoys feeling like a hamster on a wheel).

Most importantly, we'll remind you that you're not alone in this. We'll be your cheerleader, your partner in crime, and your sassy sidekick, cracking jokes and offering support along the way. Because let's face it, losing weight is way more fun with a friend!

So, ditch the fad diets and get ready to rewrite the rules. Let's embark on a journey towards a healthier, happier you, one filled with delicious food, sustainable habits, and maybe even a few laughs along the way.

The Battle of the Bulge: Understanding Why We Gain Weight (and How to Stop the Onslaught)

The dreaded bulge. It seems to appear overnight, like a stealthy ninja accumulating rent in the form of unwanted pounds. But unlike a mischievous roommate, understanding why we gain weight is the first step to taking back control and winning the battle of the bulge. So, grab your metaphorical sword and shield, because we're about to delve into the science behind weight gain and equip you with the knowledge to fight back.

Calories: The Energetic Battlefield

Imagine your body as a giant calorie-burning furnace. You throw in food (fuel), and it burns it for energy to keep you functioning. When the amount of calories you consume (the fuel you throw in) equals the amount your body burns (the energy it uses), you maintain a healthy weight. But here's where things get interesting:

- **Calorie Surplus:** If you consistently consume more calories than your body burns, it's like throwing too much fuel into the furnace. The excess gets stored as fat, leading to that pesky bulge. Think of those delicious but calorie-dense cookies you love – they taste amazing, but they also pack a serious caloric punch.
- **Calorie Deficit:** On the other hand, if you burn more calories than you consume, it's like not giving your furnace enough fuel. Your body starts tapping into stored fat for energy, leading to weight loss. This is the basic principle behind most weight loss strategies.

The Plot Thickens: Beyond the Calorie Equation

While calories play a major role, weight gain isn't just a simple math equation. There are other sneaky culprits lurking in the shadows, conspiring to expand your waistline. Let's meet these weight gain instigators:

- **Metabolism Mayhem:** Your metabolism is the rate at which your body burns calories. It's influenced by factors like age, muscle mass, and genetics. As we age, our metabolism naturally slows down, making it easier to pack on pounds. Muscle burns more calories than fat, so building muscle mass can help boost your metabolism and keep the weight off.

- **Hormonal Havoc:** Hormones play a significant role in regulating appetite, metabolism, and fat storage. Fluctuations in hormones like estrogen, testosterone, and cortisol can all contribute to weight gain. Stress, for example, can lead to increased cortisol levels, which can trigger cravings for sugary and fatty foods.
- **Sleepless Nights:** When you don't get enough sleep, your body produces more ghrelin (the hunger hormone) and less leptin (the satiety hormone). This hormonal imbalance can make you feel hungrier and lead to overeating. Aim for 7-8 hours of quality sleep each night to keep your hormones in check.
- **The Sneaky Sugar Monster:** Sugar, especially added sugar found in processed foods and sugary drinks, can wreak havoc on your weight loss goals. It spikes blood sugar levels, leading to crashes and cravings for more sugar. Over time, this can lead to insulin resistance, a condition that makes it harder for your body to burn fat for energy.
- **Liquid Calories: A Deceptive Disguise:** We often underestimate the calories we consume from beverages. Sugary sodas, juices, and even fancy coffee drinks can pack a serious caloric punch without leaving you feeling full. Stick to water, unsweetened tea, and black coffee to keep your liquid calories in check.
- **A Lifeless Lifestyle:** Sitting all day burns way fewer calories than being active. Even small bursts of movement throughout the day can make a big difference. Take the stairs instead of the elevator, park further away from your destination, or do some bodyweight exercises during your commercial breaks. Every little bit counts!
- **Mindless Munching:** We've all been there: mindlessly snacking while watching TV, scrolling through social media, or simply bored. Emotional eating, stress eating,

and boredom eating are all common culprits of weight gain. Practicing mindful eating techniques can help you become more aware of your hunger cues and avoid mindless munching.

The Weight Loss Arsenal: Arming Yourself for Success

Now that you understand the enemy (weight gain), it's time to build your arsenal for weight loss success. Here are some key strategies to keep those unwanted pounds at bay:

- **Track Your Calories:** Keeping a food journal or using a calorie tracking app can help you become more aware of your calorie intake. This can be a real eye-opener, especially when you realize how quickly those little snacks and sugary drinks can add up.
- **Become a Food Prep Pro:** Planning and prepping your meals ahead of time can help you make healthy choices and avoid unhealthy temptations when you're short on time. Pack your lunches, portion out snacks, and have healthy grab-and-go options readily available.
- **Make Friends with Fiber:** Fiber-rich foods like fruits, vegetables, and whole grains keep you feeling full for longer and can help regulate your appetite. Include plenty of fiber in your diet to feel satisfied and avoid overeating.
- **Strength Train Like a Boss:** Building muscle mass can boost your metabolism and help you burn more calories at rest. Strength training doesn't have to be intimidating — start with bodyweight exercises at home or find a workout routine you enjoy.
- **Find Your Fitness Groove:** Exercise doesn't have to be a chore. Find activities you actually enjoy, whether it's dancing, hiking, swimming, or playing a sport. When you have fun, you're more likely to stick with it in the long run.
- **Befriend Sleep:** Aim for 7-8 hours of quality sleep each night. When you're well-rested, your hormones are more balanced, and you're less likely to experience cravings or overeat.

- **Manage Stress:** Chronic stress can wreak havoc on your weight loss goals. Find healthy ways to manage stress, such as yoga, meditation, or spending time in nature.
- **Stay Hydrated:** Drinking plenty of water can help you feel full and reduce cravings. Aim for eight glasses of water per day, and adjust based on your activity level and climate.
- **Don't Skip Meals:** Skipping meals can actually backfire. It can lead to overeating later and disrupt your metabolism. Aim for regular meals and healthy snacks throughout the day to keep your blood sugar levels stable and your hunger in check.
- **Celebrate Non-Scale Victories:** Weight loss isn't just about the number on the scale. Celebrate non-scale victories like having more energy, feeling stronger, or fitting into your favorite pair of jeans. These victories can help you stay motivated on your journey.

Remember, weight loss is a marathon, not a sprint. Be patient with yourself, celebrate your progress, and don't be afraid to ask for help. With the right tools and strategies, you can win the battle of the bulge and achieve your health and fitness goals.

Metabolism Mayhem: Is It Really Ruining Your Weight Loss Dreams?

Ah, metabolism. That mysterious force often blamed for sluggish weight loss or seemingly effortless skinny jeans on our co-worker, Brenda. But what exactly is metabolism, and is it truly the villain in our weight loss stories? Buckle up, because we're about to debunk some myths and shed light on this fascinating (and sometimes misunderstood) bodily process.

Metabolism 101: The Burning Furnace Within

Imagine your body as a giant furnace, constantly burning fuel (calories) to keep you functioning. This burning process is your metabolism. It's responsible for everything from keeping your heart beating and your brain firing to regulating your body temperature and helping you digest food. The more efficiently your metabolism works, the more calories you burn at rest, even while you're Netflix binging (although maybe try some jumping jacks during commercials for an extra boost!).

Several factors influence your metabolic rate, including:

- **Basal Metabolic Rate (BMR):** This is the number of calories your body burns at rest, just to keep your basic functions going. It accounts for about 60-70% of your total daily calorie expenditure. Factors like your age, gender, muscle mass, and genetics all play a role in your BMR.
- **Thermic Effect of Food (TEF):** This is the energy your body uses to digest and absorb food. Protein requires more energy to digest than carbs or fats, so a protein-rich diet can slightly boost your metabolism.
- **Physical Activity Energy Expenditure (PAEE):** This is the energy you burn through physical activity, from your daily walks to intense workouts. The more active you are, the more calories you burn and the higher your overall metabolic rate.

The Age-Old Myth: Does Metabolism Slow Down With Age?

It's true that your BMR tends to decrease slightly with age. This is partly due to a decrease in muscle mass, which burns more calories than fat. However, the decline is often much smaller than people think. Studies suggest a decrease of around 2-3% per decade after age 30.

So, while age might play a role, it's not an excuse to throw in the weight loss towel. Focusing on building muscle mass, staying active, and making smart food choices can all help counteract the age-related decline in metabolism.

Metabolism Myths Debunked!

The internet is full of misinformation about metabolism. Here are some common myths we need to bust:

- **Myth #1: Eating Spicy Food Boosts Metabolism Significantly:** While spicy food might temporarily raise your heart rate and body temperature, the effect on your overall metabolism is minimal. Don't drown your food in hot sauce just yet.
- **Myth #2: Certain "Metabolism-Boosting" Supplements Are Magic Bullets:** Unfortunately, there's no magic pill for a permanently revved-up metabolism. Most "metabolism boosters" are ineffective and often have unsubstantiated claims. Focus on building healthy habits instead.
- **Myth #3: Skipping Meals Speeds Up Metabolism:** This is a recipe for disaster. Skipping meals can actually slow down your metabolism as your body goes into starvation mode and tries to conserve energy. Aim for regular meals and healthy snacks throughout the day.
- **Myth #4: Eating Small Frequent Meals Keeps Your Metabolism Fired Up:** While there isn't enough evidence to suggest one specific meal frequency is superior for everyone, the focus should be on overall calorie intake and healthy eating patterns. Don't get caught up in rigid meal schedules – find what works best for you.

The Truth About Muscle Mass and Metabolism

Muscle is metabolically active tissue. It burns more calories at rest than fat, so building muscle mass can give your metabolism a natural boost. Strength training doesn't have to be intimidating –

start with bodyweight exercises at home or find a workout routine you enjoy. Even small increases in muscle mass can make a significant difference in your overall calorie burn.

Optimizing Your Metabolic Engine

Here are some actionable tips to keep your metabolism functioning optimally:

- **Strength Train Regularly:** As mentioned before, building muscle is a great way to boost your metabolism. Aim for at least two to three strength training sessions per week.
- **Move Your Body:** Physical activity of any kind helps burn calories. Find activities you enjoy, whether it's dancing, swimming, hiking, or playing a sport. Aim for at least 150 minutes of moderate-intensity exercise or 75 minutes of vigorous-intensity exercise per week.
- **Eat a Balanced Diet:** Focus on whole, unprocessed foods like fruits, vegetables, whole grains, and lean protein. These foods provide essential nutrients and keep you feeling full longer, which can help regulate your appetite and prevent overeating.
- **Stay Hydrated:** Drinking plenty of water can help with digestion, reduce cravings, and even slightly boost your metabolism. Aim for eight glasses of water per day, and adjust based on your activity level and climate.
- **Get Enough Sleep:** Chronic sleep deprivation can disrupt hormones that regulate appetite and metabolism. Aim for 7-8 hours of quality sleep each night.
- **Manage Stress:** Chronic stress can lead to increased cortisol levels, a hormone that can promote weight gain and negatively impact metabolism. Find healthy ways to manage stress, such as yoga, meditation, or spending time in nature.

Remember, metabolism is just one piece of the weight loss puzzle. By focusing on healthy habits, a balanced diet, and regular exercise, you can create a sustainable approach to weight loss and keep your body's natural burning furnace functioning optimally.

Sugar Shock! How Sweet Treats Can Leave You Bitter (and Bigger)

Let's face it, folks, sugar is everywhere. It lurks in our favorite snacks, drinks, and even seemingly healthy-sounding products. It whispers sweet nothings in our ears, promising a burst of energy and a momentary taste of bliss. But the truth is, sugar can be a sneaky saboteur in our weight loss journey, leaving us feeling sluggish, cranky, and maybe a few pounds heavier. Buckle up, because we're about to delve into the science of sugar and explore how to outsmart this sweet villain.

The Deceptive Allure of Sugar

Sugar, particularly added sugar found in processed foods and sugary drinks, provides a quick hit of energy. When we consume sugar, our bodies break it down into glucose, a simple sugar that enters our bloodstream. This rise in blood sugar triggers the release of insulin, a hormone that helps our cells take up glucose for energy.

Here's where things get interesting:

- **The Blood Sugar Rollercoaster:** That initial sugar rush is often followed by a crash as blood sugar levels plummet. This crash can leave you feeling tired, irritable, and craving more sugar to get back to that initial high. It's a vicious cycle that can wreak havoc on your energy levels and appetite.

- **The Hunger Hormone Havoc:** Sugar can also disrupt the production of hormones like leptin (the satiety hormone) and ghrelin (the hunger hormone). This can lead to increased hunger and cravings, making it harder to stick to a healthy diet.

- **The Insulin Resistance Blues:** Over time, a diet high in added sugar can lead to insulin resistance. This means your body becomes less efficient at using insulin to move glucose into cells. This can further disrupt your blood sugar balance and contribute to weight gain.

Sugar in Disguise: The Hidden Culprits

Sugar isn't always as obvious as a bowl of candy. It can be hiding in seemingly healthy foods like yogurt, salad dressings, and even whole-wheat bread. Here are some clever ways sugar disguises itself:

- **High Fructose Corn Syrup:** This is a common sweetener found in processed foods and beverages. It's even more damaging than table sugar because it can be more readily stored as fat in the liver.
- **Agave Nectar:** While touted as a healthier alternative, agave nectar is still high in fructose and can have similar effects on your blood sugar as table sugar.
- **Fruit Juices:** While fruit provides essential nutrients, fruit juice is often loaded with concentrated sugar and lacks the fiber found in whole fruit. This can lead to a quick blood sugar spike and crash.

Breaking Free from the Sugar Trap

So, how do we break free from the clutches of sugar and reclaim control of our health? Here are some actionable steps:

- **Become a Label Detective:** Read food labels carefully. Look for added sugars and be mindful of serving sizes. Don't be fooled by misleading marketing claims.
- **Make Friends with Whole Foods:** Focus on whole, unprocessed foods like fruits, vegetables, whole grains, and lean protein. These foods are naturally lower in sugar and provide essential nutrients that keep you feeling full and satisfied.
- **Sweeten Naturally:** Instead of added sugar, try natural sweeteners like stevia, monk fruit extract, or a sprinkle of cinnamon. These options provide sweetness without the blood sugar spike.
- **Go for the Whole Fruit:** Choose whole fruit over fruit juice. Whole fruit provides fiber, which helps slow down the absorption of sugar into the bloodstream.
- **Plan Your Snacks:** Don't be caught unprepared when hunger strikes. Have healthy snacks readily available, like fruits and vegetables with a bit of nut butter, yogurt with berries, or homemade trail mix.

- **Mindful Indulgence:** It's okay to enjoy occasional treats. The key is moderation and mindful eating. Savor your treat, eat it slowly, and pair it with a healthy option like fruit or nuts.
- **Detox Your Taste Buds:** The more sugar you consume, the sweeter your taste buds crave. Gradually reduce added sugar in your diet, and you'll find yourself appreciating the natural sweetness of whole foods.
- **Cook More at Home:** Cooking at home gives you control over the ingredients. You can limit added sugar and create healthy and delicious meals.
- **Find Healthy Alternatives:** Craving something sweet? Try a smoothie made with frozen fruit and yogurt, baked apples with a sprinkle of cinnamon, or dark chocolate with a high cacao content (70% or higher).

Remember, sugar doesn't have to be the enemy. By being mindful of your sugar intake, making smart food choices, and finding healthy alternatives, you can break free from the sugar trap and achieve your health and weight loss goals.

The Label Labyrinth: Deciphering Food Labels Without Getting Lost in the Fine Print

Standing in the grocery aisle, surrounded by a sea of colorful packaging and confusing labels, can feel like navigating a labyrinth. You want to make healthy choices, but deciphering food labels can be like trying to decode a secret code. Fear not, fellow food adventurer! This chapter is your guide to navigating the label labyrinth, equipping you with the knowledge to make informed choices and fuel your body for success.

The Label Breakdown: Unveiling the Mysteries

Food labels are packed with information, but let's be honest, some of it can feel like a foreign language. Here's a breakdown of the key components to focus on:

- **Serving Size:** This is crucial! All the calorie and nutrient information listed is based on this serving size. Don't be fooled by packages that seem small – sometimes one serving is actually half the package! Pay attention to the number of servings per container and adjust your calculations accordingly.
- **Calories:** This tells you how much energy the food provides. Use this information to stay within your daily calorie goals for weight loss or maintenance.
- **Calories from Fat:** This tells you how many calories come from fat in the serving. It's helpful to keep saturated and trans fats low for optimal health.
- **Total Fat, Saturated Fat, Trans Fat:** These tell you the total amount of fat, the amount of saturated fat (unhealthy), and the amount of trans fat (very unhealthy) in the serving. Aim to limit saturated and trans fats as much much as possible.
- **Cholesterol:** This tells you the amount of cholesterol in the serving. While dietary cholesterol can impact overall cholesterol levels, focus on limiting saturated and trans fats for a bigger impact.

- **Sodium:** This tells you the amount of sodium (salt) in the serving. Too much sodium can contribute to high blood pressure. Aim for products lower in sodium, especially if you're watching your blood pressure.
- **Total Carbohydrates, Dietary Fiber, Sugars:** This section breaks down the carbs into total carbs, dietary fiber (good for you!), and sugars (including added sugars). Focus on whole grains and high-fiber options for sustained energy and gut health. Limit added sugars for overall health.
- **Protein:** This tells you the amount of protein in the serving. Protein is essential for building and repairing tissues. Aim for protein sources throughout the day for satiety and muscle building.
- **Vitamins and Minerals:** This section lists essential vitamins and minerals like Vitamin D, Calcium, and Iron. These are crucial for various bodily functions. Aim for a variety of foods to get a full spectrum of essential nutrients.

Beyond the Basics: Decoding Marketing Claims

Food labels are often plastered with marketing claims designed to grab your attention. Here's how to approach them with a critical eye:

- **"Natural":** This term doesn't necessarily mean healthy. A product can be natural and still be high in sugar or unhealthy fats.
- **"Low-Fat" or "Fat-Free":** These products may be lower in fat, but they might be compensated for with added sugar or unhealthy fillers.
- **"Sugar-Free" or "No Added Sugar":** These can be misleading. The product may still contain naturally occurring sugars or artificial sweeteners.
- **"Healthy Choice" or "Good Source of":** These claims are often subjective. Check the overall nutrient content for a more complete picture.

Pro Tips for Label Literacy

Here are some additional tips to become a label-reading pro:

- **Compare Similar Products:** Compare the labels of similar products to find the option with the most favorable nutrient profile for your needs.
- **Don't Be Afraid to Flip the Package:** The ingredients list is typically displayed in descending order by weight. The first few ingredients make up the bulk of the product.
- **Focus on Whole Foods:** When possible, choose whole foods that don't require a label. Fruits, vegetables, whole grains, and lean protein sources are generally good bets.
- **Use Resources:** Utilize online resources and apps to help you decipher labels and understand the health implications of different ingredients.

Remember, food labels are a valuable tool, but they shouldn't be the sole factor in your food choices. Use your knowledge to make informed decisions, but also prioritize overall dietary patterns and focus on enjoying a variety of healthy and delicious foods.

Friend, Not Foe: Making Food Your Ally in Weight Management

Portion Patrol: Mastering the Art of Mindful Eating Without Feeling Deprived

Ah, portion control. Those two little words can strike fear into the hearts of even the most determined weight loss warriors. We picture tiny, sad salads and measuring out every almond. But fear not, portion patrol doesn't have to be a joyless exercise in deprivation. In this chapter, we'll explore the art of mindful eating, helping you develop healthy habits and make smart choices without feeling like you're constantly saying "no" to delicious food.

The Portion Problem: Why We Overeat

Let's face it, portion sizes have ballooned over the years. Supersized drinks, restaurant meals that could feed a small family, and those ubiquitous "family-sized" packages at the grocery store – it's no wonder we often struggle with portion control. Here are some reasons why we might overeat:

- **External Cues:** We're bombarded with cues to eat more, from oversized portions to tempting advertising.
- **Mindless Munching:** We eat while distracted (think scrolling through social media) and don't pay attention to internal hunger cues.
- **Emotional Eating:** We turn to food for comfort, stress relief, or boredom, leading to overconsumption.
- **Habits:** We're conditioned to finish everything on our plate or clear the serving dish, even if we're no longer hungry.

Mindful Eating: The Key to Portion Control

Mindful eating is all about developing a conscious awareness of your eating habits. It's about slowing down, savoring your food, and tuning into your body's hunger and fullness cues. Here are some tips to cultivate mindful eating:

- **Practice Gratitude:** Before you dig in, take a moment to appreciate your food. Consider where it came from, the effort it took to prepare it, and the nourishment it will provide.
- **Eat Slowly and Savor Each Bite:** Put down your phone, turn off the TV, and focus on the act of eating. Chew your food thoroughly and savor the flavors.
- **Listen to Your Body:** Pay attention to your hunger cues. Start eating when you're slightly hungry and stop when you're comfortably full, not stuffed.
- **Use Smaller Plates:** Using a smaller plate can create the illusion of a larger portion, making you feel more satisfied with less food.
- **Distinguish Cravings from Hunger:** True hunger is a gradual feeling, while cravings are often intense and sudden. Ask yourself if you're truly hungry or if there's another reason you're reaching for food.
- **Plan Your Meals and Snacks:** Having healthy options readily available can prevent mindless snacking and help you stick to portion control.
- **Don't Skip Meals:** Skipping meals can lead to overeating later. Aim for regular meals and healthy snacks throughout the day.

Portion Control Strategies: Putting It All Together

Now that you understand mindful eating, here are some practical strategies for portion control:

- **Pre-portion Snacks:** Divide snacks like nuts, yogurt, or fruits into individual containers to avoid mindlessly grabbing handfuls.
- **Measure and Portion:** Use measuring cups and spoons, especially for calorie-dense foods like nuts, seeds, and salad dressings.
- **Downsize Your Dinnerware:** Opt for smaller plates and bowls to trick your brain into feeling satisfied with less food.
- **Leftovers Are Your Friend:** When dining out, ask for a take-home box right away. This helps you avoid

overindulging and ensures you have a healthy portion for another meal.

- **Focus on Nutrient Density:** Prioritize nutrient-rich foods like fruits, vegetables, and whole grains. These foods are filling and keep you satisfied for longer.
- **Drink Plenty of Water:** Water can help curb hunger pangs and make you feel fuller sooner. Aim for eight glasses of water per day, and adjust based on your activity level and climate.

Remember, portion control is a journey, not a destination. There will be bumps along the road, but with practice and mindful eating techniques, you can develop healthy habits that support your weight loss goals and overall well-being.

Pantry Power: Stocking Your Kitchen for Weight Loss Success (and Avoiding the Hangry Monster)

Ah, the pantry. That magical (or sometimes not-so-magical) space where temptation lurks alongside the potential for healthy choices. When your pantry is stocked with nutritious goodies, you're setting yourself up for success in your weight loss journey. But with aisles overflowing with processed options, building a weight-loss friendly pantry can feel overwhelming. Fear not, fellow food warriors! This chapter will be your guide to pantry power, equipping you with the knowledge to create a haven of healthy staples that will keep you fueled and your taste buds happy.

The Pantry Purge: Bidding Farewell to Bulky Bullies

Before you embark on your pantry stocking spree, it's time for a purge. Let's tackle those unhealthy items that might derail your good intentions. Here's what to ditch:

- **Sugary Cereals:** Swap sugary cereals for high-fiber options like oatmeal, whole-wheat flakes, or unsweetened shredded wheat.
- **Refined Grains:** Replace white bread, pasta, and rice with whole-wheat alternatives. Whole grains are higher in fiber and keep you feeling fuller for longer.
- **Processed Snacks:** Chips, cookies, crackers – these are often loaded with unhealthy fats, sodium, and added sugars. Opt for healthier snack alternatives like nuts, seeds, or dried fruit.
- **Sugary Drinks:** Soda, juice, and sugary sports drinks are loaded with empty calories. Stock your fridge with water, unsweetened tea, and sparkling water instead.
- **Healthy-ish Imposters:** Granola bars, fat-free cookies, and diet chips often contain hidden sugars and unhealthy fats. Read labels carefully and choose whole, unprocessed foods whenever possible.

The Pantry Powerhouse: Must-Have Staples for Weight Loss Success

Now for the fun part – building your weight-loss friendly pantry! Here are some essential staples to keep on hand:

- **Whole Grains:** Stock up on brown rice, quinoa, whole-wheat pasta, and whole-wheat bread. These provide sustained energy and essential nutrients.
- **Beans and Lentils:** These are a vegetarian powerhouse, packed with protein and fiber. They're perfect for adding to soups, salads, and stews.
- **Canned Fish:** Canned tuna, salmon, and sardines are excellent sources of lean protein and healthy fats. They're also shelf-stable and convenient for quick meals.
- **Dried Fruits and Nuts:** A handful of nuts and seeds provides a satisfying dose of healthy fats, protein, and fiber. Choose unsalted and unsweetened varieties for optimal health benefits. Dried fruits are a great source of natural sweetness, but be mindful of portion sizes.
- **Healthy Oils:** Keep a variety of healthy oils like olive oil, avocado oil, or canola oil on hand for cooking and salad dressings.
- **Spices and Herbs:** Spices and herbs add flavor to your food without adding extra calories or sodium. Experiment with different combinations to create delicious and healthy meals.
- **Condiments with a Kick:** Ditch the sugary sauces and dressings. Opt for options like salsa, low-sodium soy sauce, or balsamic vinegar.
- **Healthy Sweeteners:** If you have a sweet tooth, keep a small amount of a natural sweetener like honey, maple syrup, or stevia on hand. Use them sparingly and be mindful of portion sizes.

Pantry Power Plays: Putting It All Together

Here are some additional tips to get the most out of your pantry:

- **Plan Your Meals:** Planning your meals ahead of time helps you avoid unhealthy impulse purchases and ensures you have the ingredients on hand for healthy options.

- **Cook More at Home:** Cooking at home gives you control over the ingredients you use. You can limit unhealthy fats, added sugars, and sodium.
- **Don't Fear Frozen:** Frozen fruits and vegetables are a great option to keep on hand. They're flash-frozen at peak ripeness, locking in nutrients.
- **Read Labels:** Just because something is labeled "healthy" doesn't mean it is. Always read labels carefully and be mindful of added sugars and sodium content.
- **Make Healthy Swaps:** Craving something salty? Reach for air-popped popcorn instead of chips. Need a sweet treat? Try a piece of fruit with a dollop of nut butter instead of cookies.

Remember, your pantry is your ally in your weight loss journey. By stocking up on healthy staples and planning your meals, you can avoid the hangry monster and make healthy choices a breeze.

Conquering the Cravings: Outsmarting Your Body's Battle Cry for Bad Decisions

Ah, cravings. Those insistent whispers (or sometimes shrieks) from our bodies that can derail even the most well-intentioned weight loss plans. They seem to appear out of nowhere, urging us to reach for that extra slice of pizza or a pint of ice cream. But fear not, fellow warriors! In this chapter, we'll explore the science behind cravings, equip you with strategies to outsmart them, and develop healthy coping mechanisms to keep you on track towards your weight loss goals.

The Craving Culprits: Why We Want What We Can't Have (Sometimes)

Cravings are complex and influenced by a variety of factors, including:

- **Blood Sugar Swings:** When blood sugar levels drop, our bodies crave quick sources of energy, often in the form of sugary or high-carbohydrate foods.
- **Hormonal Fluctuations:** Hormonal changes, like those experienced during menstruation or PMS, can trigger cravings for specific foods.
- **Emotional Eating:** We often turn to food for comfort, stress relief, or boredom. This emotional connection can lead to cravings for unhealthy options.
- **Memories and Associations:** Certain foods or smells can trigger memories and emotional associations. The sight of your grandma's famous cookies might trigger a craving, even if you're not physically hungry.
- **Food Addiction:** In some cases, cravings can be a sign of food addiction, a complex condition characterized by a loss of control over eating.

Outsmarting the Craving Monster: Taking Back Control

While cravings can be powerful, there are ways to outsmart them and make healthy choices. Here are some strategies to keep your cravings in check:

- **Identify Your Triggers:** Pay attention to what triggers your cravings. Are you stressed? Bored? Tired? Once you identify your triggers, you can develop coping mechanisms to deal with them in healthy ways.
- **Don't Deprive Yourself Completely:** Deprivation can often lead to intense cravings and binge eating. Allow yourself occasional treats in moderation, but focus on healthy options most of the time.
- **Plan Your Meals and Snacks:** Don't leave yourself feeling famished. Aim for regular meals and healthy snacks throughout the day to keep your blood sugar levels stable and cravings at bay.
- **Stay Hydrated:** Dehydration can sometimes mimic hunger pangs. Drinking plenty of water can help curb cravings and keep you feeling full.
- **Get Enough Sleep:** Chronic sleep deprivation can disrupt hormones that regulate appetite and cravings. Aim for 7-8 hours of quality sleep each night.
- **Manage Stress:** Stress can be a major trigger for cravings. Find healthy ways to manage stress, such as yoga, meditation, or spending time in nature.
- **Healthy Distractions:** When a craving hits, distract yourself with a healthy activity you enjoy. Go for a walk, listen to music, or read a book.
- **Mindful Eating:** Slow down and pay attention to your body's hunger cues. Eat slowly and savor your food. This can help you feel satisfied with less food and reduce cravings.
- **Don't Keep Trigger Foods Around:** If certain foods are your biggest craving culprits, avoid keeping them in the house. Opt for healthier alternatives that won't derail your progress.

Craving Hacks: Swapping Unhealthy Options for Healthy Satisfiers

Sometimes, a craving just won't quit. Here are some healthy swaps to satisfy your cravings without sabotaging your weight loss goals:

- **Craving Something Sweet:** Instead of sugary treats, reach for fruits with natural sweetness, a piece of dark chocolate, or a small serving of frozen yogurt with berries.
- **Craving Something Salty:** Opt for air-popped popcorn with a sprinkle of herbs, baked kale chips, or a handful of roasted chickpeas instead of chips or pretzels.
- **Craving Something Crunchy:** Munch on raw vegetables with hummus, roasted nuts and seeds, or a homemade trail mix with whole-grain cereal and dried fruit instead of potato chips or fried snacks.
- **Craving Something Creamy:** Try Greek yogurt with fruit and a drizzle of honey, a smoothie made with fruits and vegetables, or a bowl of oatmeal with nut butter instead of ice cream or creamy desserts.
- **Craving Comfort Food:** Make a healthier version of your comfort food classic. Swap white pasta for whole-wheat noodles in your mac and cheese, or use lean ground turkey in your chili.

Remember, conquering cravings is a journey, not a destination. There will be times when cravings win, but don't let that discourage you. Get back on track with your next meal and celebrate your small victories. With practice and the strategies outlined in this chapter, you can develop healthy coping mechanisms and keep cravings from derailing your weight loss goals.

From Bland to Grand: Delicious and Healthy Recipes That Won't Make You Want to Cry

Let's face it, healthy eating sometimes gets a reputation for being bland and boring. Salads every day? No thank you! But fear not, fellow food adventurers! This chapter is your gateway to a world of delicious and healthy recipes that will tantalize your taste buds and keep you on track with your weight loss goals.

We'll explore a variety of recipes to suit different dietary needs and preferences. From protein-packed breakfasts to veggie-loaded dinners and satisfying snacks, you'll find inspiration to create meals that are both nutritious and delicious.

Breakfast Powerhouses: Fueling Your Day the Healthy Way

- **Scrambled Eggs with Spinach and Feta:** This protein-packed option is ready in minutes. Sauté some spinach with chopped onions and garlic, then scramble eggs with feta cheese and spices. Serve on a whole-wheat toast for a complete and satisfying breakfast.

- **Overnight Oats with Berries and Chia Seeds:** Perfect for busy mornings, overnight oats are a healthy and delicious way to start your day. Combine rolled oats, yogurt, milk, chia seeds, and your favorite fruits in a jar and refrigerate overnight. In the morning, you'll have a grab-and-go breakfast packed with fiber and protein.

- **Smoothie Bowl Extravaganza:** Blend your favorite fruits, yogurt, spinach, and protein powder for a smoothie base. Pour it into a bowl and top with a variety of goodies like granola, nut butter, sliced banana, or chia seeds. It's a fun and customizable way to enjoy a nutritious breakfast.

Light and Flavorful Lunch Options to Keep You Going

- **Quinoa Salad with Grilled Chicken and Roasted Vegetables:** This protein- and veggie-packed salad is perfect for a satisfying lunch. Cook quinoa, grill chicken breast, and roast your favorite vegetables. Toss everything together with a light vinaigrette dressing.

- **Lentil Soup with Whole-Wheat Bread:** This hearty soup is a budget-friendly and nutritious lunch option. Lentils are packed with protein and fiber, while vegetables add essential vitamins and minerals. Serve with a slice of whole-wheat bread for a complete meal.
- **Tuna Salad with Whole-Wheat Pita Bread:** Ditch the mayo-laden tuna salad! Combine canned tuna with chopped celery, red onion, Greek yogurt, lemon juice, and spices. Serve it on whole-wheat pita bread for a light and flavorful lunch.

Dinner Delights: Nourishing Your Body and Pleasing Your Palate

- **Salmon with Roasted Asparagus and Quinoa:** Salmon is a great source of lean protein and healthy fats. Roast asparagus alongside quinoa for a complete and satisfying meal. Season everything with herbs and spices for added flavor.
- **Turkey Chili with Whole-Wheat Cornbread:** This chili is a hearty and comforting dinner option. Use lean ground turkey, black beans, kidney beans, and your favorite chili spices. Serve it with a side of whole-wheat cornbread for a delicious and satisfying meal.
- **Vegetarian Stir-Fry with Brown Rice:** This is a quick and easy way to get your daily dose of vegetables. Choose a variety of colorful veggies like broccoli, carrots, peppers, and snap peas. Stir-fry them with tofu or tempeh for a plant-based protein option. Serve over brown rice for a complete meal.

Snack Time Satisfaction: Healthy Nibbles to Keep Hunger at Bay

- **Apple Slices with Almond Butter:** This classic combination is a healthy and satisfying snack. Apples provide fiber and natural sweetness, while almond butter adds protein and healthy fats.
- **Greek Yogurt with Berries:** Greek yogurt is a great source of protein and calcium. Top it with your favorite berries for a delicious and nutritious snack.

- **Carrot Sticks with Hummus:** Carrots are a good source of beta-carotene, while hummus provides protein and healthy fats. This is a perfect snack for dipping.
- **Homemade Trail Mix:** Make your own trail mix with nuts, seeds, dried fruits, and whole-grain cereal. This is a customizable and satisfying snack option.
- **Roasted Edamame:** Edamame is a great source of plant-based protein and fiber. Roast them with a sprinkle of sea salt for a healthy and delicious snack.

Remember, healthy eating doesn't have to be boring! With a little creativity and exploration, you can find delicious and satisfying recipes that support your weight loss goals. Experiment with different flavors and ingredients to discover your new favorite healthy meals.

This is just a taste of the many delicious and healthy recipes available. With a little creativity and exploration, you can find endless options to keep your meals interesting and your taste buds happy.

Cooking Up Fun: Making Meal Prep a Breeze (and Maybe Even Enjoyable)

Let's face it, the thought of meal prep can feel like another chore on your already overflowing to-do list. Visions of bland chicken breasts and steamed broccoli might dance in your head, leaving you feeling defeated before you even begin. But fear not, fellow warriors! This chapter is your guide to transforming meal prep from a dreaded task into a fun and efficient way to stay on track with your weight loss goals.

We'll explore tips and tricks to make meal prep a breeze, saving you time and money throughout the week. We'll also show you how to inject some creativity and flavor into your meals, ensuring they're not only healthy but also delicious.

The Meal Prep Mindset: Setting Yourself Up for Success

Before diving into grocery lists and containers, let's shift your mindset around meal prep. Here's how to approach it with a positive outlook:

- **Think of it as Self-Care:** Meal prep is an investment in your health and well-being. Having healthy meals readily available removes the temptation of unhealthy choices when you're short on time.
- **Plan for Success:** Dedicate a specific time each week for meal prep. This could be a Sunday afternoon session or a quick prep session in the evenings after work. Planning ahead ensures you have the ingredients and time needed.
- **Focus on Efficiency:** Choose recipes with overlapping ingredients to minimize chopping and prep time. Utilize kitchen appliances like a food processor or slow cooker to save time and effort.
- **Get Creative!:** Meal prep doesn't have to be boring! Explore different flavor profiles and cuisines to keep your meals interesting. Experiment with spices, herbs, and sauces to add variety.

The Meal Prep Arsenal: Must-Have Tools and Equipment

To make meal prep a smooth operation, here are some essential tools to have on hand:

- **Sharp Knives:** A good quality chef's knife and a paring knife will make chopping and prepping ingredients a breeze.
- **Cutting Boards:** Invest in a sturdy cutting board to protect your countertops and make chopping safer.
- **Storage Containers:** Choose a variety of airtight containers to store your prepped meals and snacks. Look for containers that are microwave-safe and dishwasher-safe for added convenience.
- **Sheet Pans:** Sheet pans are perfect for roasting vegetables, baking proteins, or reheating prepped meals.
- **Food Processor:** A food processor can save you a ton of time chopping and prepping vegetables.
- **Slow Cooker:** A slow cooker allows you to toss in ingredients in the morning and have a delicious, cooked meal ready by dinner time. Perfect for busy schedules!

The Meal Prep Masterplan: A Step-by-Step Guide

Now that you've got the right mindset and tools, let's dive into the meal prep process:

1. **Pick Your Day:** Dedicate a specific day or block of time each week for meal prep. Consistency is key to making this a sustainable habit.
2. **Plan Your Meals:** Choose recipes that are healthy, delicious, and easy to prep in advance. Consider your dietary needs and preferences when making your selections.
3. **Make a Grocery List:** Create a detailed list of all the ingredients you'll need for your chosen recipes. Sticking to your list helps avoid impulse purchases and keeps you on budget.
4. **Shop Smart:** Head to the grocery store armed with your list and stick to it! Consider buying pre-cut vegetables or pre-cooked grains to save time on prepping.
5. **Prepping Like a Pro:** Wash and chop your vegetables, cook your grains, and prepare your proteins according to

your recipes. Portion everything out into your storage containers for easy grab-and-go meals throughout the week.

6. **Label It Up:** Label your containers with the meal name and the date to avoid any confusion during the week.
7. **Storing for Freshness:** Store your prepped meals in the refrigerator or freezer depending on how far in advance you've prepped them. Most cooked meals will stay fresh in the refrigerator for 3-4 days.
8. **Reheating and Enjoying:** When it's meal time, simply grab your container and reheat it according to the instructions. Add a touch of freshness with chopped herbs or a squeeze of lemon juice before serving.

Meal Prep Magic: Tips and Tricks for Success

Here are some additional hacks to take your meal prep game to the next level:

- **Double Up on Recipes:** Cook a larger batch of a recipe and freeze half for another week. This saves you time in the long run.
- **Get the Family Involved:** Delegate tasks like washing vegetables or setting the table to make meal prep a family affair.
- **Clean as You Go:** Wash your dishes and clean up as you go to avoid a giant mess at the end of your prep session.
- **Portion Control is Key:** Pre-portioning your meals helps with mindful eating and prevents overeating.
- **Don't Be Afraid to Leftover-fy:** Get creative with leftovers! Use leftover roasted vegetables in an omelette or leftover chicken in a salad.
- **Variety is the Spice of Life:** Choose a variety of recipes throughout the week to keep your meals interesting and prevent taste bud burnout.

Remember, meal prep is a skill that takes practice. Don't get discouraged if your first attempt isn't perfect. With a little planning and these helpful tips, you can transform meal prep into a time-saving and healthy habit that supports your weight loss goals. Now go forth and conquer the kitchen!

Moving It, Moving It: Exercise Without the Excuses

Finding Your Fitness Groove: Discovering Activities You Actually Don't Hate

The dreaded "E" word. Exercise. For many, it conjures images of dusty treadmills, crowded gyms, and sheer boredom. But fear not, fellow adventurers! This chapter is your guide to discovering movement that feels good for your body and sparks joy in your soul. We'll explore a variety of activities beyond the traditional gym routine, helping you find your fitness groove and make physical activity a sustainable part of your weight loss journey.

Shifting Your Mindset: From Obligation to Exploration

The first step is to ditch the negative associations with exercise. Instead of viewing it as a chore, approach it with an open mind and a sense of exploration. Here's how to reframe your thinking:

- **Focus on How You Feel:** Instead of focusing on weight loss, prioritize how exercise makes you feel. Aim for activities that leave you energized, empowered, and happy.
- **Celebrate Movement:** Our bodies were meant to move! Find joy in the simple act of physical activity, whether it's a brisk walk in nature or dancing to your favorite music.
- **It Doesn't Have to Be All or Nothing:** Don't feel pressured to spend hours in the gym. Even small bursts of activity throughout the day can make a big difference. Take the stairs instead of the elevator, park further away from your destination, or do some bodyweight exercises during your commercial breaks.
- **Find Your Tribe:** Exercising with a friend or joining a group fitness class can add a social element and boost motivation. There's a fitness community for everyone, so find yours!

Exploring the Fitness Universe: Activities Beyond the Gym Walls

The world of fitness is vast and varied. Here are some ideas to get you started:

- **Team Sports:** Join a recreational sports team for a fun and social way to get active. Options abound, from basketball and soccer to volleyball and flag football.
- **Dance it Out:** From Zumba to salsa to ballroom dancing, there's a dance style for everyone. Put on your favorite music and let loose!
- **Martial Arts:** Martial arts like karate, taekwondo, or kickboxing offer a great workout that combines physical activity with self-defense skills.
- **Rock Climbing:** Indoor climbing gyms offer a challenging and fun workout that builds strength and coordination.
- **Hiking and Biking:** Explore nature and get some exercise at the same time. Hiking and biking are fantastic ways to get your heart rate up and enjoy the fresh air.
- **Swimming:** Swimming is a low-impact, full-body workout that's easy on your joints. It's perfect for people of all ages and fitness levels.
- **Yoga and Pilates:** These mind-body practices combine physical postures with breathwork to improve flexibility, strength, and core stability.
- **High-Intensity Interval Training (HIIT):** HIIT workouts alternate between short bursts of intense activity and recovery periods. They're a time-efficient way to get a great workout in a short amount of time.
- **Home Workouts:** No gym membership required! There are countless free workout routines available online that you can do from the comfort of your own home. Utilize bodyweight exercises, resistance bands, or free weights to create a challenging workout.
- **Active Games:** Turn playtime into exercise time! Play tag with your kids, have a dance party in your living room, or challenge them to a game of jump rope.
- **Household Chores:** Believe it or not, even household chores can get your heart rate up. Crank up some music and turn cleaning into a mini-workout.

Remember, the key is to find activities you enjoy. If you're having fun, you're more likely to stick with it in the long run. Don't be afraid to experiment and try different things until you find your fitness sweet spot.

Making It a Habit: Building Consistency in Your Fitness Routine

Here are some tips to help you make physical activity a regular part of your life:

- **Start Small and Gradually Increase:** Don't try to do too much too soon. Begin with shorter workouts and gradually increase the duration and intensity as you get stronger.
- **Schedule Your Workouts:** Treat your workouts like important appointments and schedule them into your calendar. This will help you stay committed.
- **Find an Accountability Partner:** Enlist a friend or family member to join you on your fitness journey. Having someone to hold you accountable can make a big difference.
- **Track Your Progress:** Keep track of your workouts and celebrate your milestones. Seeing your progress can be a great motivator.
- **Reward Yourself:** Set small goals and reward yourself for achieving them. This will help you stay motivated and on track.
- **Listen to Your Body:** Take rest days when you need them and don't push yourself too hard. It's important to avoid injuries.

Embrace the Journey: Fitness is a lifelong pursuit, not a quick fix. There will be ups and downs along the way, but the most important thing is to keep moving. Find activities you enjoy, celebrate your progress, and don't be afraid to have fun! With dedication and a positive attitude, you can discover the joy of movement and make physical activity a cornerstone of your healthy lifestyle.

Building a Sustainable Routine: Making Exercise a Habit That Sticks

Congratulations! You've explored the world of healthy eating, conquered cravings, and discovered the joy of movement. Now comes the crucial part: making these positive changes a sustainable part of your life. This chapter delves into the science of habit formation and equips you with strategies to ensure your exercise routine sticks around for the long haul.

The Habit Loop: Understanding How Habits Form

Our brains rely on habits for efficiency. They automate repetitive behaviors, freeing up mental space for more complex tasks. The habit loop, a concept popularized by Charles Duhigg, explains the three key steps involved in forming a habit:

1. **Cue:** This is the trigger that initiates the behavior. It could be a specific time of day, a certain location, or an emotional state.
2. **Routine:** This is the actual behavior itself – your workout in this case.
3. **Reward:** This is the positive reinforcement that your brain receives after completing the behavior. It could be the feeling of accomplishment, increased energy levels, or simply the satisfaction of sticking to your plan.

Making Exercise a Habit: Strategies for Sticking with It

Understanding the habit loop empowers you to create an exercise routine that sticks. Here are some strategies to implement:

- **Identify Your Cues:** What triggers you to want to exercise? Is it seeing your workout clothes laid out in the morning? Hearing your favorite workout playlist? Once you know your cues, you can leverage them to your advantage.
- **Stack Habits:** Pair your new exercise routine with an existing habit. For example, if you always drink coffee in the morning, lace up your shoes and do a quick workout before your cup of joe.

- **Make it Convenient:** Choose activities that fit your schedule and lifestyle. If you're short on time, opt for shorter, high-intensity workouts. Consider home workouts if commuting to the gym is a barrier.
- **Set SMART Goals:** Set Specific, Measurable, Achievable, Relevant, and Time-bound goals. Aim for small, incremental improvements that you can celebrate along the way.
- **Find an Exercise Buddy:** Having an accountability partner can boost motivation and make workouts more fun.
- **Track Your Progress:** Keep track of your workouts in a journal or app. Seeing your progress can be a powerful motivator.
- **Reward Yourself:** Celebrate your milestones! Reward yourself for sticking to your routine, but choose healthy and non-food-related rewards like a new workout outfit or a relaxing massage.
- **Focus on Progress, Not Perfection:** There will be days when you miss a workout or don't feel like exercising. Don't beat yourself up! Just get back on track with your next workout.
- **Make it Enjoyable:** This is crucial! Choose activities you genuinely enjoy. If you hate running, don't force yourself to do it. Find something that makes you feel good and look forward to your workouts.

Building a Sustainable Routine: Beyond the Basics

Here are some additional tips to consider as you build your sustainable routine:

- **Be Flexible:** Life happens. Be prepared to adjust your workout schedule as needed, but don't let a missed workout derail your entire routine.
- **Listen to Your Body:** Rest days are essential for recovery. Don't push yourself too hard and pay attention to your body's signals.
- **Embrace Variety:** Incorporate different activities into your routine to keep things interesting and prevent boredom.

- **Celebrate Non-Scale Victories:** Focus on how exercise makes you feel, not just the numbers on the scale. Celebrate increased energy levels, improved sleep, or greater strength.
- **Find Inspiration:** Surround yourself with positive influences. Follow fitness accounts on social media, read inspiring stories, or listen to motivational podcasts.

Remember, building a sustainable exercise routine is a journey, not a destination. There will be setbacks along the way, but with dedication and the strategies outlined in this chapter, you can create a habit of movement that supports your health and well-being for the long haul. Embrace the process, celebrate your victories, and enjoy the journey to a healthier, happier you!

The Taming of the Gym: Conquering Your Gym Intimidation (and Those Lunks Who Hog the Machines)

Ah, the gym. For some, it's a haven of fitness inspiration and iron-pumping bliss. For others, it's a land of intimidating grunts, unfamiliar equipment, and the lurking fear of judgement. But fear not, fellow warriors! This chapter is your guide to conquering your gym intimidation and transforming it into a place of empowerment and progress.

We'll tackle the common anxieties associated with the gym, equip you with strategies to navigate the space with confidence, and even show you how to deal with those gym etiquette offenders who hog the machines (without resorting to fisticuffs).

Why We Fear the Gym: Unveiling the Intimidation Monster

Let's be honest, gyms can be intimidating. Here are some common reasons why people feel apprehensive:

- **Fear of Being Judged:** We all have that nagging voice in our heads telling us everyone is staring and critiquing our every move.
- **Feeling Out of Place:** Gyms can be filled with experienced gym-goers who seem to know exactly what they're doing. This can make newcomers feel lost and out of place.
- **Unfamiliarity with Equipment:** The rows of machines and free weights can be overwhelming, especially if you don't know how to use them properly.
- **The "Lunk" Factor:** Let's face it, some gym users have perfected the art of hogging machines, leaving others waiting and feeling frustrated.

Slaying the Intimidation Dragon: Strategies for Gym Confidence

Here's how to transform your gym experience from anxiety-inducing to awesome:

- **Shift Your Mindset:** Focus on your own goals and forget about everyone else. The gym is for you, not for them.
- **Start Small and Celebrate Progress:** Don't try to do too much too soon. Begin with a manageable workout routine and celebrate your milestones, big or small.

- **Embrace the Learning Curve:** It's okay not to know how to use every piece of equipment. Ask a trainer for guidance or find instructional videos online.
- **Find Your Tribe:** Consider working out with a friend or joining a group fitness class. Having a support system can boost motivation and make the gym a more social experience.
- **Invest in a Few Personal Training Sessions:** A few sessions with a personal trainer can teach you proper form, create a personalized workout plan, and boost your confidence in the gym.
- **Dress for Success:** Wear workout clothes that make you feel comfortable and confident. Looking good can help you feel good.
- **Focus on Your Workout:** Put on your headphones, tune out the distractions, and focus on getting the most out of your workout.

Conquering the "Lunk" Factor: Gym Etiquette for Everyone

Let's address the inconsiderate gym users who disrupt the flow for everyone else. Here are some etiquette tips to ensure a smooth and respectful gym experience for all:

- **Wipe Down Equipment After Use:** No one wants to use a sweaty machine. Wipe down your equipment after each use with a disinfectant wipe.
- **Don't Hog Machines:** If you're resting between sets, be courteous and let others waiting use the equipment. Finish your sets, then take your rest periods off the machine.
- **Re-Rack Your Weights:** Don't leave weights scattered around the gym floor. Put them back where they belong after use.
- **Be Mindful of Others:** Avoid slamming weights, yelling excessively, or monopolizing benches for stretching while others wait.
- **Ask Permission Before Working In:** If someone is already using a piece of equipment, politely ask if you can work in with them.

- **Be Aware of Your Surroundings:** Maintain spatial awareness and avoid blocking walkways or having your swinging weights impede others.

Remember, a little gym etiquette goes a long way. By following these tips, you can create a more positive and respectful environment for everyone.

The Gym: Your Gateway to Fitness

The gym doesn't have to be a scary place. With the right mindset and strategies, you can transform it into a supportive environment for reaching your fitness goals. So take a deep breath, conquer your intimidation, and embrace the gym as your personal playground for health and empowerment.

The Joy of Movement: Exploring Fun Exercise Options That Don't Feel Like Work.

Let's face it, traditional exercise routines can feel like a chore. The thought of endless sets on the treadmill or lifting weights can leave you feeling demotivated before you even begin. But fear not, fellow adventurers! This chapter is your guide to discovering movement that feels good for your body and sparks joy in your soul. We'll explore a variety of activities beyond the gym walls, helping you find the fun in fitness and make physical activity a sustainable part of your weight loss journey.

Reframing Exercise: From Obligation to Exploration

The first step is to ditch the negative associations with exercise. Instead of viewing it as a chore, approach it with an open mind and a sense of exploration. Here's how to reframe your thinking:

- **Focus on How You Feel:** Instead of focusing solely on weight loss, prioritize how exercise makes you feel. Aim for activities that leave you energized, empowered, and happy.
- **Celebrate Movement:** Our bodies were meant to move! Find joy in the simple act of physical activity, whether it's dancing to your favorite music or a brisk walk in nature.
- **Every Step Counts:** Don't feel pressured to spend hours exercising. Even small bursts of activity throughout the day can make a big difference. Take the stairs instead of the elevator, park further away from your destination, or do some bodyweight exercises during commercial breaks.

Unleashing Your Inner Child: Rediscovering the Fun of Movement

Remember how much fun you used to have playing games and being active as a child? Reconnect with that playful spirit and explore activities that bring you joy:

- **Dance it Out:** From Zumba to salsa to ballroom dancing, there's a dance style for everyone. Put on your favorite music and let loose!

- **Join a Recreational Sports Team:** Basketball, soccer, volleyball, or even a friendly game of flag football - team sports offer a fun and social way to get active.
- **Hit the Trails:** Hiking and biking are fantastic ways to explore nature and get your heart rate up. Breathe in the fresh air and enjoy the scenery.
- **Embrace the Water:** Swimming is a low-impact, full-body workout that's easy on your joints. There's a reason why water activities are so popular!
- **Channel Your Inner Warrior:** Martial arts like karate, taekwondo, or kickboxing provide a challenging workout that builds strength, coordination, and self-defense skills.
- **Challenge Yourself:** Rock climbing offers a physical and mental challenge that builds strength, coordination, and problem-solving skills. Indoor climbing gyms provide a safe and controlled environment to get started.
- **Get Groovy with Yoga or Pilates:** These mind-body practices combine physical postures with breathwork to improve flexibility, strength, and core stability. Many variations cater to different fitness levels.
- **Embrace the HIIT Wave:** High-Intensity Interval Training (HIIT) workouts alternate between short bursts of intense activity and recovery periods. They're a time-efficient way to get a great workout in a short amount of time.
- **Home is Your Gym:** No gym membership required! There are countless free workout routines available online that you can do from the comfort of your own home. Utilize bodyweight exercises, resistance bands, or free weights to create a challenging workout.
- **Active Gaming:** Turn playtime into exercise time! Play active video games with motion sensors that get you moving, or have a dance party in your living room with your favorite music.
- **Make it a Family Affair:** Involve your family in your fitness journey! Go for bike rides together, play tag in the park, or have a family dance competition.

- **Household Chores Can Be Fun (Ish):** Believe it or not, even household chores can get your heart rate up. Crank up some music and turn cleaning into a mini-workout session.

Remember, the key is to find activities you enjoy. If you're having fun, you're more likely to stick with it in the long run. Don't be afraid to experiment and try different things until you find your fitness sweet spot.

Keeping the Fun Alive: Strategies for Maintaining Exercise Enjoyment

Here are some tips to ensure your exercise routine stays enjoyable:

- **Mix it Up:** Don't get stuck in a rut! Try different activities to keep things interesting and prevent boredom.
- **Find an Exercise Buddy:** Enlist a friend or family member to join you on your fitness journey. Having someone to exercise with can add a social element and boost motivation.
- **Reward Yourself:** Set small goals and reward yourself for achieving them. This will help you stay motivated and on track.
- **Track Your Progress:** Seeing your progress, even small improvements, can be a great motivator. Keep a log of your workouts or use a fitness app to track your activity.
- **Listen to Your Body:** Don't push yourself too hard and take rest days when you need them. It's important to avoid injuries.

Embrace the Journey: Fitness is a lifelong pursuit, not a quick fix. There will be ups and downs along the way, but the most important thing is to keep moving. Find activities you enjoy, celebrate your progress, and don't be afraid to have fun! With a positive attitude and a playful spirit, you can transform exercise from a chore into a joyful celebration of movement.

Battling Boredom: Keeping Your Workouts Fresh and Exciting.

Congratulations! You've conquered your initial exercise hurdle and discovered the joy of movement. But even the most enthusiastic fitness newbie can fall victim to the dreaded "workout rut." The same routine day in and day out can become monotonous, leading to a decline in motivation and ultimately, a stalled weight loss journey. Fear not, fellow warriors! This chapter equips you with strategies to keep your workouts fresh, exciting, and effective, ensuring you stay on track and reach your goals.

The Boredom Battleground: Why Workouts Become Monotonous

There are several reasons why workouts can become boring:

- **Routine Repetition:** Doing the same exercises day after day can lead to a lack of challenge and a plateau in progress.
- **Lack of Variety:** Sticking to just one type of exercise (e.g., treadmill running) neglects other muscle groups and can become stale.
- **Predictability:** Knowing exactly what to expect from your workout every time can zap the element of surprise and excitement.

Slaying the Boredom Dragon: Strategies for Keeping Workouts Fresh

Here are some tips to inject new life into your exercise routine:

- **Mix Up Your Modes of Movement:** Incorporate a variety of activities into your week. Try weightlifting one day, a HIIT class the next, and a yoga session on the third.
- **Target Different Muscle Groups:** Don't neglect any muscle group! Design your workouts to target all major muscle groups throughout the week.
- **Progress, Not Perfection:** Gradually increase the intensity, duration, or difficulty of your workouts to keep challenging yourself and seeing results.

- **Embrace the Great Outdoors:** Take your workout outside for a change of scenery! Go for a run in the park, hike a new trail, or do bodyweight exercises at a local park.
- **Join a Group Fitness Class:** Group fitness classes offer a fun and social way to exercise. There's a class for everyone, from Zumba and dance to spinning and bootcamp.
- **Invest in Online Workouts:** Numerous free and paid online workout resources offer a vast library of routines you can do from the comfort of your home.
- **Interval Training is Your Friend:** HIIT workouts or other interval training methods alternate between high-intensity bursts and recovery periods, keeping your workouts dynamic and efficient.
- **Strength Train for More Than Just Definition:** Strength training not only builds muscle but also boosts your metabolism and helps you burn more calories at rest.
- **Technology Can Be Your Ally:** Download fitness apps to track your workouts, discover new routines, or find workout partners.
- **Challenge Yourself with New Activities:** Step outside your comfort zone and try something new! Take a rock climbing class, learn a new dance style, or go kayaking.
- **Find Inspiration Online:** Social media can be a great source of fitness inspiration. Follow fitness accounts, watch workout videos, and get motivated by others' journeys.
- **Plan Fitness Themed Adventures:** Turn your weekend getaway into a fitness adventure! Hike a new mountain range, go for a bike ride through a scenic vineyard, or take a surf lesson at the beach.
- **Reward Yourself for Trying New Things:** Incentivize yourself to explore new activities by setting small goals and rewarding yourself for achieving them.
- **Listen to Your Body:** Don't push yourself to the point of burnout. If you're not feeling a particular activity, take a break or choose something else.

- **Focus on the Fun Factor:** Remember, exercise should be enjoyable! Choose activities you genuinely find fun so you look forward to your workouts.

Building a Sustainable Routine: Variety is Key

By incorporating variety into your routine, you'll keep your workouts interesting, challenge your body in new ways, and prevent plateaus in your progress. Here are some additional tips for building a sustainable and varied routine:

- **Plan Your Workouts:** Schedule your workouts in advance and treat them like important appointments. This will help you stay committed.
- **Set Realistic Goals:** Set SMART goals (Specific, Measurable, Achievable, Relevant, and Time-bound) that are challenging but achievable. Celebrate your progress along the way.
- **Find an Accountability Partner:** Having a workout buddy or joining a fitness community can provide support and motivation.
- **Track Your Progress:** Keeping track of your workouts helps you see your progress and stay motivated. Use a workout journal, app, or wearable fitness tracker.
- **Listen to Your Body and Take Rest Days:** Rest and recovery are essential for muscle growth and preventing injuries. Don't push yourself too hard, and schedule rest days into your routine.

The Final Boss: Maintaining Long-Term Motivation

Remember, staying motivated is a journey, not a destination. There will be days when you don't feel like exercising. Here are some tips to keep yourself going:

- **Focus on How You Feel:** Instead of just focusing on weight loss, remember how exercise makes you feel – energized, empowered, and confident.
- **Visualize Your Goals:** Keep your fitness goals in mind and visualize yourself achieving them. This can be a powerful motivator.

- **Celebrate Non-Scale Victories:** Focus on more than just the numbers on the scale. Celebrate increased energy levels, improved sleep, or greater strength.
- **Find Inspiration:** Surround yourself with positive influences. Follow fitness accounts, read inspiring stories, or listen to motivational podcasts.
- **Remember Why You Started:** Reflect on your initial reasons for starting your fitness journey. What are you hoping to achieve? Reconnecting with your "why" can reignite your motivation.

Embrace the Journey: Fitness is a lifelong pursuit, not a quick fix. There will be ups and downs along the way, but the most important thing is to keep moving. By incorporating variety into your routine, finding activities you enjoy, and staying motivated, you can transform exercise into a sustainable habit that supports your health and well-being for the long haul. So keep exploring, keep moving, and celebrate your journey to a healthier, happier you!

Mind Over Matter: Conquering the Mental Game of Weight Loss

Silence the Inner Critic: Taming Your Negative Self-Talk and Building Body Confidence.

Ah, the inner critic. That nagging voice in our heads that whispers doubts, insecurities, and negativity, especially when it comes to our bodies. This chapter equips you with tools to silence that critic, cultivate self-acceptance, and build unshakeable body confidence – a crucial pillar on your weight loss journey and beyond.

The Inner Critic's Grip: Understanding Negative Self-Talk

We all have an inner critic, a voice shaped by societal expectations, past experiences, and negative self-beliefs. This voice often manifests as negative self-talk, which can sound like:

- "I'll never look good in a swimsuit."
- "I'm so weak and out of shape."
- "Everyone else at the gym looks so much better than me."

These negative thoughts can be incredibly damaging, hindering our motivation, progress, and overall well-being.

Taming the Inner Critic: Strategies for Building Body Confidence

Here's how to silence the inner critic and cultivate self-love:

- **Identify Your Triggers:** Pay attention to situations that trigger your negative self-talk. Is it looking in the mirror? Seeing others at the gym? Once you identify the triggers, you can develop strategies to address them.
- **Challenge Your Negative Thoughts:** Don't accept your negative thoughts as truth. Challenge them with more realistic and positive statements. For example, instead of "I'll never look good in a swimsuit," try "I'm getting stronger and healthier, and that's what matters."
- **Focus on Progress, Not Perfection:** Celebrate your progress, no matter how small. Focus on how far you've come instead of fixating on what you perceive as flaws.

- **Practice Gratitude:** Take time each day to appreciate your body for all it allows you to do. It carries you, helps you experience the world, and deserves your respect and gratitude.
- **Affirmations Can Be Powerful:** Use positive affirmations to counter negative self-talk. Repeat positive statements about yourself daily, such as "I am strong," "I am worthy," or "I am becoming healthier every day."
- **Embrace Body Positivity:** Surround yourself with positive influences and messages. Follow body-positive accounts on social media, read books and articles promoting self-acceptance, and challenge unrealistic beauty standards.
- **Focus on How You Feel, Not How You Look:** Shift your focus from appearance to how exercise makes you feel. Do you have more energy? Feel stronger? Sleep better? Celebrate these non-scale victories.
- **Treat Yourself with Kindness:** Talk to yourself the way you would talk to a friend. Would you ever tell a friend they're weak or out of shape? Be kind and compassionate towards yourself.
- **Visualize Success:** Imagine yourself achieving your goals and feeling confident in your body. Visualization can be a powerful tool for self-belief.
- **Celebrate Non-Appearance Milestones:** Did you run a farther distance this week? Lift a heavier weight? Celebrate these achievements that showcase your improving strength and fitness.
- **Focus on What You Can Control:** You can't control everything, like genetics or societal beauty standards. But you can control your effort, attitude, and the choices you make. Focus on what's within your power.
- **Reward Yourself for Positive Self-Talk:** When you catch yourself challenging negative thoughts and replacing them with positive affirmations, reward yourself! This reinforces the positive behavior.
- **Seek Support:** Don't be afraid to talk to a therapist or counselor if negative self-talk is significantly impacting

your life. They can provide professional guidance and support for developing healthy self-esteem.

Building Body Confidence: It's a Journey, Not a Destination

Building body confidence is a journey, not a destination. There will be good days and bad days. But by incorporating these strategies into your daily life, you can gradually silence the inner critic and cultivate self-acceptance. Here are some additional tips:

- **Wear Clothes That Make You Feel Good:** Look and feel your best in clothes that flatter your figure and make you feel confident.
- **Focus on Your Strengths:** What do you love about your body? Maybe it's your strong legs, your radiant smile, or your infectious laugh. Highlight your strengths and focus on what makes you unique.
- **Compare Yourself to You, Not Others:** Social media can be a breeding ground for comparison. Avoid comparing your body to others'. Focus on your own journey and celebrate your individual progress.
- **Focus on Health, Not Weight:** Ultimately, health is more important than weight. Focus on making healthy choices that nourish your body and make you feel good.
- **Forgive Yourself for Setbacks:** Everyone has setbacks. Don't beat yourself up if you have a bad day or indulge in a treat. Forgive yourself, get back on track, and keep moving forward.

Remember, you are worthy of love and respect, regardless of your size or shape. By silencing the inner critic and cultivating body confidence, you'll not only improve your weight loss journey but also build a stronger foundation for overall well-being and happiness.

Stress Less, Weigh Less: Managing Stress for Healthy Eating and Exercise Habits

Chronic stress can wreak havoc on your weight loss journey. It disrupts your hormones, increases cravings for unhealthy foods, and zaps your motivation to exercise. This chapter explores the connection between stress and weight management, and equips you with effective strategies to manage stress and create a healthier, happier you.

The Stress-Weight Connection: How Stress Sabotages Your Goals

Stress is a natural response to challenging situations. It releases hormones like cortisol, which can:

- **Increase Appetite:** Cortisol stimulates cravings for sugary and fatty foods, often leading to unhealthy choices.
- **Promote Fat Storage:** Cortisol can lead to increased belly fat storage, making weight loss more challenging.
- **Disrupt Sleep:** Stress can disrupt sleep patterns, leaving you feeling tired and lacking the energy needed for healthy eating and exercise.
- **Decrease Motivation:** Chronic stress can zap your motivation to cook healthy meals and exercise, hindering your weight loss efforts.

Breaking the Cycle: Effective Stress Management Techniques

Now that you understand how stress can sabotage your goals, let's explore techniques to manage stress effectively:

- **Identify Your Stressors:** The first step is to identify the things that cause you stress. Is it work deadlines, financial worries, or relationship issues? Once you know what triggers your stress, you can develop coping mechanisms.
- **Relaxation Techniques:** Practice relaxation techniques such as deep breathing exercises, meditation, progressive muscle relaxation, or yoga. These techniques can help calm your mind and body during stressful times.
- **Mindfulness Practice:** Mindfulness involves focusing on the present moment without judgment. Mindfulness

practices like meditation can help you manage stress and improve your overall well-being.

- **Get Enough Sleep:** Aim for 7-8 hours of quality sleep each night. Adequate sleep helps regulate hormones, improves mood, and boosts energy levels, making you better equipped to handle stress.
- **Exercise Regularly:** Exercise is a natural stress reliever. Regular physical activity releases endorphins, which have mood-boosting effects and can help combat stress.
- **Healthy Eating Habits:** While comfort food may seem tempting during stressful times, focus on nourishing your body with whole, unprocessed foods. This will provide you with sustained energy and support your stress management efforts.
- **Connect with Loved Ones:** Social support is crucial for managing stress. Spend time with loved ones who make you feel happy and supported.
- **Learn to Say No:** Don't overload your schedule or take on more than you can handle. Learn to politely decline commitments that will add unnecessary stress to your life.
- **Set Boundaries:** Establish healthy boundaries at work and in personal relationships. This helps you manage your time and reduce stress.
- **Make Time for Fun:** Schedule time for activities you enjoy, whether it's reading, spending time in nature, or listening to music. Taking breaks and having fun helps reduce stress and boosts overall well-being.
- **Challenge Negative Thoughts:** Stressful situations can often lead to negative self-talk. Challenge these thoughts and replace them with positive affirmations.
- **Seek Professional Help:** If stress feels overwhelming and is significantly impacting your daily life, consider seeking professional help from a therapist or counselor. They can provide guidance and support for developing healthy coping mechanisms.

Building a Stress-Management Toolkit

The key to managing stress effectively is to develop a personal toolkit of techniques that work for you. Experiment with different approaches and find what helps you feel calm and centered. Here are some additional tips for building your toolkit:

- **Create a Relaxing Routine:** Establish a relaxing bedtime routine to wind down before sleep. This could involve taking a warm bath, reading a book, or practicing light stretches.
- **Spend Time in Nature:** Studies show that spending time in nature can significantly reduce stress levels. Go for a walk in the park, hike in the woods, or simply sit outside and soak up the sunshine.
- **Practice Gratitude:** Taking time each day to appreciate the good things in your life can help shift your perspective and reduce stress. Keep a gratitude journal or simply take a few minutes each day to reflect on what you're thankful for.
- **Laugh it Off:** Laughter is a powerful stress reliever. Watch a funny movie, spend time with someone who makes you laugh, or read a humorous book.
- **Listen to Calming Music:** Soothing music can have a relaxing effect on the mind and body. Create a playlist of calming music to listen to when you're feeling stressed.
- **Digital Detox:** Take regular breaks from social media and electronic devices. The constant stimulation from technology can contribute to stress. Schedule time to disconnect and recharge.

Remember, managing stress is an ongoing process. There will be times when stress levels rise, but by incorporating these strategies into your life, you'll be better equipped to handle what comes your way. A calmer, more stress-free you will find it much easier to make healthy choices, stay motivated, and achieve your weight loss goals.

Sleep for Success: How Catching Zzz's Can Help You Reach Your Weight Loss Goals

Ever feel like you're working out religiously and eating clean, yet the weight loss seems stagnant? Sleep, often the most neglected factor, might be the missing puzzle piece. This chapter explores the powerful link between sleep and weight management, and equips you with strategies to achieve restful sleep, ultimately propelling you towards your weight loss goals.

The Sleep-Weight Connection: Why Sleep Matters for Weight Loss

When you don't get enough sleep, a symphony of hormones gets disrupted, impacting your weight management efforts in several ways:

- **Increased Appetite:** Sleep deprivation disrupts leptin (the satiety hormone) and ghrelin (the hunger hormone) levels, leading to increased appetite and cravings for unhealthy, high-calorie foods.
- **Decreased Metabolism:** Sleep deprivation can slow down your metabolism, the rate at which your body burns calories. This makes it harder to lose weight and keep it off.
- **Impaired Impulse Control:** When you're sleep-deprived, your willpower weakens, making it more difficult to resist unhealthy temptations and cravings.
- **Increased Stress:** Lack of sleep can elevate stress hormones like cortisol, which can promote fat storage, particularly around the belly.

The Power of Sleep: How Restful Nights Support Weight Loss

Adequate sleep (around 7-8 hours per night for most adults) offers a multitude of benefits for weight management:

- **Appetite Regulation:** Proper sleep helps regulate leptin and ghrelin levels, promoting feelings of fullness and reducing cravings.
- **Boosted Metabolism:** Adequate sleep can support a healthy metabolism, aiding in efficient calorie burning.

- **Improved Impulse Control:** When you're well-rested, you have better willpower and can make healthier food choices.
- **Stress Reduction:** Quality sleep helps combat stress, keeping cortisol levels in check and preventing stress-induced weight gain.
- **Increased Physical Activity Levels:** Feeling well-rested gives you more energy to engage in physical activity, a crucial component of weight loss.

Building a Sleep Sanctuary: Strategies for Restful Nights

Creating a sleep-conducive environment and establishing a relaxing bedtime routine are essential for achieving quality sleep. Here are some tips:

- **Optimize Your Sleep Environment:** Ensure your bedroom is dark, quiet, cool, and clutter-free. Invest in blackout curtains, an earplug mask, and a comfortable mattress and pillows.
- **Develop a Relaxing Bedtime Routine:** Wind down before bed with calming activities like taking a warm bath, reading a book, or practicing relaxation techniques like deep breathing or meditation.
- **Establish a Sleep Schedule:** Go to bed and wake up at consistent times each day, even on weekends. This helps regulate your body's natural sleep-wake cycle.
- **Limit Screen Time Before Bed:** The blue light emitted from electronic devices can disrupt sleep patterns. Avoid screens for at least an hour before bedtime.
- **Create a Sleep-Promoting Diet:** Limit caffeine and alcohol intake, especially in the evening, as they can interfere with sleep quality. Avoid heavy meals close to bedtime.
- **Regular Exercise:** Regular physical activity promotes better sleep, but avoid strenuous workouts too close to bedtime.
- **Address Underlying Issues:** If you suspect you have a sleep disorder like sleep apnea, consult a doctor for diagnosis and treatment.

Making Sleep a Priority: Investing in Your Overall Health

Prioritizing sleep is an investment in your overall health and well-being. By incorporating these strategies and creating healthy sleep habits, you'll not only improve your weight loss efforts but also experience a multitude of benefits, including increased energy levels, improved mood, and enhanced cognitive function.

The Power of Patience: Celebrating Milestones and Avoiding Discouragement.

The road to weight loss is a marathon, not a sprint. There will be victories and setbacks, moments of excitement and frustration. This chapter equips you with the power of patience, the resilience to navigate challenges, and the art of celebrating milestones – all crucial for staying motivated and reaching your weight loss goals.

The Patience Paradox: Embracing the Journey

In our fast-paced world, we often crave instant results. But weight loss is a journey, not a destination. It takes time, dedication, and a healthy dose of patience to achieve lasting results. Here's why patience is key:

- **Sustainable Habits Take Time:** Building healthy habits takes time and consistent effort. Don't get discouraged if you don't see results overnight.
- **Weight Loss is a Gradual Process:** Aim for a healthy weight loss of 1-2 pounds per week. Slow and steady wins the race!
- **Setbacks are Inevitable:** Everyone experiences setbacks along the way. The key is to learn from them, get back on track, and keep moving forward.

Cultivating Patience: Strategies for Staying Motivated

Here's how to cultivate patience and stay motivated on your weight loss journey:

- **Set Realistic Goals:** Setting unrealistic goals can lead to disappointment and discouragement. Focus on achievable, measurable goals that celebrate progress.
- **Focus on Non-Scale Victories:** The scale isn't the only measure of success. Celebrate non-scale victories like increased energy levels, improved sleep, stronger muscles, or fitting into your favorite clothes again.
- **Find Inspiration:** Surround yourself with positive influences. Follow inspiring weight loss journeys on social

media, read motivational books, or listen to podcasts about health and wellness.
- **Reward Yourself:** Celebrate your milestones, big or small! Rewarding yourself with non-food rewards can keep you motivated and reinforce positive behavior.
- **Visualize Success:** Take time to visualize yourself achieving your weight loss goals. See yourself feeling confident, healthy, and happy. Visualization can be a powerful tool for motivation.
- **Practice Gratitude:** Take time each day to appreciate your body for all it allows you to do. Gratitude fosters a positive mindset and helps you stay focused on your goals.
- **Find a Support System:** Having a support system of friends, family, or a weight loss group can be invaluable. They can provide encouragement, hold you accountable, and celebrate your successes.
- **Focus on Progress, Not Perfection:** There will be days when you slip up. Don't beat yourself up! Forgive yourself, learn from the experience, and recommit to your goals.
- **Enjoy the Process:** Focus on making healthy choices that nourish your body and make you feel good. Find activities you enjoy, whether it's cooking healthy meals, trying new workout routines, or spending time outdoors. This will make your weight loss journey more sustainable and enjoyable.

The Art of Celebration: Recognizing and Rewarding Your Achievements

Celebrating your milestones, big or small, is an essential part of staying motivated. Here's how to effectively celebrate your achievements:
- **Public Recognition (Optional):** If comfortable, share your achievements with friends and family. Their support and encouragement can be a great motivator.
- **Experiences Over Things:** Opt for experience-based rewards over food or material possessions. This could

involve a relaxing massage, a weekend getaway, or a new workout outfit.

- **Align Rewards with Your Values:** Choose rewards that align with your overall health and wellness goals. For example, a spa day or a cooking class focused on healthy recipes.
- **Make It Memorable:** Take photos or document your milestones in a journal. This will serve as a reminder of your progress and how far you've come.

Remember, patience is a muscle that strengthens with practice. By incorporating these strategies, you can cultivate patience, stay motivated, and celebrate your achievements along the way. This will empower you to navigate challenges, overcome setbacks, and ultimately reach your weight loss goals.

Building a Support System: Finding Your Cheerleaders and Ditching the Debbie Downers

The road to weight loss can feel lonely at times. But you don't have to go it alone! Having a strong support system can be the difference between success and failure. This chapter explores the importance of surrounding yourself with positive influences, finding your cheerleaders, and identifying negativity that can hinder your progress.

The Power of Support: Why You Need Your Cheer Squad

A supportive network of friends, family, or a weight loss group can provide invaluable benefits on your weight loss journey:

- **Motivation and Encouragement:** A support system can keep you motivated, especially on challenging days. They'll celebrate your victories and encourage you during setbacks.
- **Accountability:** Knowing someone is holding you accountable can make you more likely to stick to your goals.
- **Shared Experiences:** Being around others who understand your struggles and triumphs can be incredibly comforting and motivating.
- **Knowledge Sharing:** You can swap healthy recipe ideas, workout routines, and tips with your support system, fostering a sense of community.
- **Emotional Support:** A supportive network can provide a safe space to vent frustrations, celebrate victories, and receive emotional support throughout your journey.

Building Your Dream Team: Identifying Your Ideal Support System

The ideal support system is comprised of individuals who:

- **Are Positive and Encouraging:** Surround yourself with people who believe in you and celebrate your progress.
- **Respect Your Goals:** Find people who understand and support your weight loss goals, even if they don't share the same journey.

- **Offer Encouragement Without Judgment:** Your support system should uplift you without making you feel pressured or judged.
- **Lead by Positive Example:** Ideally, your support system includes people who also prioritize healthy habits, but this isn't always necessary.
- **Are Trustworthy and Respectful:** Confide in people you trust to keep your struggles and triumphs confidential.

Identifying and Eliminating Debbie Downers

Not everyone will be supportive of your weight loss journey. Some people, often unintentionally, can be negativity influences, also known as "Debbie Downers." Here's how to identify and minimize their impact:

- **The Skeptic:** This person doubts your ability to succeed and may make discouraging comments.
- **The Saboteur:** This person may tempt you with unhealthy foods or encourage you to skip workouts.
- **The Competitor:** This person may try to downplay your achievements or make the journey about them.
- **The Unhelpful Commentator:** This person may make unsolicited comments about your weight or appearance, even if they mean well.

Strategies for Dealing with Negativity

- **Limit Contact:** If someone consistently drains your motivation, limit your interactions with them.
- **Set Boundaries:** Communicate your goals and boundaries to those who might be unintentionally negative.
- **Focus on Your Goals:** Don't let negativity derail you. Remind yourself of your "why" and stay focused on your own journey.
- **Find Positivity Elsewhere:** Surround yourself with positive influences who uplift and encourage you.

Building Your Cheer Squad: Where to Find Your Support System

There are many ways to build a strong support system:

- **Friends and Family:** Talk to your loved ones about your goals and enlist their support.

- **Weight Loss Groups:** Joining a weight loss group connects you with others on a similar journey, fostering a sense of community and shared experience.
- **Online Support Groups:** Online communities and forums offer support and encouragement from a wider range of people.
- **Accountability Partners:** Find a friend or family member to be your accountability partner. Regularly check in with each other and motivate each other.
- **Fitness Professionals:** Personal trainers, nutritionists, and therapists can provide guidance, support, and motivation throughout your journey.

Remember, a supportive network is a powerful tool for success. By surrounding yourself with positive influences and minimizing negativity, you'll create a foundation for motivation, encouragement, and ultimately, weight loss achievement.

Conclusion: Maintaining the Magic: How to Keep the Weight Off and Live a Healthy, Happy Life.

Congratulations! You've reached the conclusion of this comprehensive guide. You've learned valuable strategies for weight loss, built a foundation for healthy habits, and discovered the importance of self-love and a positive mindset. But remember, weight loss is just the beginning. This chapter equips you with the tools to maintain your weight loss, embrace a healthy lifestyle, and live a happy, fulfilling life.

From Weight Loss to Lifestyle Change: Shifting Your Focus

Think of your weight loss journey not as a temporary fix, but as a springboard to a healthier, happier lifestyle. Here's how to make the transition:

- **Focus on How You Feel:** Instead of just focusing on the number on the scale, prioritize how healthy habits make you feel – energized, empowered, and confident.
- **Make Healthy Habits Sustainable:** Focus on creating sustainable lifestyle changes you can maintain in the long term. Don't deprive yourself; find healthy alternatives you enjoy.
- **Celebrate Non-Scale Victories:** Continue to celebrate non-scale victories like improved sleep, increased strength, or better fitting clothes.
- **Maintenance is a Journey:** Remember, maintaining your weight loss is an ongoing process. There will be ups and downs, but don't see a setback as a failure. View it as a learning experience and get back on track.

Building a Healthy Life: Habits for Long-Term Success

Here are some habits to integrate into your life for long-term success:

- **Regular Physical Activity:** Aim for at least 150 minutes of moderate-intensity exercise or 75 minutes of vigorous-intensity exercise per week. Find activities you enjoy and make them a regular part of your routine.

- **Healthy Eating Habits:** Focus on a balanced diet rich in fruits, vegetables, whole grains, and lean protein. Limit processed foods, sugary drinks, and unhealthy fats.
- **Mindful Eating:** Practice mindful eating, paying attention to hunger and fullness cues. Eat slowly and savor your food.
- **Prioritize Sleep:** Aim for 7-8 hours of quality sleep each night. Adequate sleep is crucial for overall health and weight management.
- **Stress Management:** Develop healthy coping mechanisms to manage stress effectively. Techniques like yoga, meditation, and deep breathing can be helpful.
- **Regular Check-Ups:** Schedule regular check-ups with your doctor to monitor your health and progress.
- **Embrace Self-Care:** Make time for activities that nourish your mind, body, and soul. This could include spending time in nature, reading, or pursuing hobbies you enjoy.

Remember, you are not alone on this journey. Surround yourself with positive influences, seek support when needed, and celebrate your achievements, big and small. By prioritizing your health and well-being, you can maintain your weight loss, live a healthy and fulfilling life, and radiate confidence from the inside out.

Bonus Chapter: Life Happens: Navigating Weight Loss Through Holidays, Vacations, and Other Curveballs.

Life throws curveballs. Holidays, vacations, birthdays, stressful work periods – these events can disrupt your routines and threaten to derail your weight loss progress. But fear not, warriors! This bonus chapter equips you with strategies to navigate these challenges, minimize setbacks, and stay on track towards your health and wellness goals.

The Curveball Effect: How Life Events Can Impact Weight Loss

Here's how unexpected events can impact your weight loss journey:

- **Disrupted Routines:** Holidays and vacations often involve changes in eating habits, exercise routines, and sleep patterns.
- **Increased Stress:** Stressful events can lead to emotional eating and unhealthy coping mechanisms.
- **Temptations Galore:** Holidays and celebrations often involve tempting treats and social pressures to indulge.
- **Travel Challenges:** Maintaining healthy habits can be difficult when traveling due to limited access to healthy food options and exercise routines.

Strategies for Hitting a Home Run: Conquering Weight Loss Challenges

Here's how to navigate life's curveballs and minimize their impact on your progress:

- **Plan Ahead:** Anticipate upcoming challenges and develop strategies to address them. Research healthy restaurant options for vacations or plan healthy snacks to bring on trips.
- **Be Flexible:** Life happens! Don't beat yourself up if your routine gets disrupted. Focus on getting back on track as soon as possible.

- **Focus on Progress, Not Perfection:** There will be times when you indulge or miss a workout. Don't let setbacks define you. Remember, progress over perfection is key.
- **Healthy Alternatives:** Find healthy alternatives to your favorite holiday treats. Focus on enjoying smaller portions and making healthier choices whenever possible.
- **Maintain Some Routine:** Even on vacations or busy days, try to maintain some semblance of your routine. Squeeze in a quick workout or pack healthy snacks to avoid unhealthy choices on the go.
- **Portion Control:** Practice mindful eating and portion control, even when faced with tempting treats. Enjoy smaller portions and savor the flavors.
- **Don't Skip Meals:** Skipping meals can lead to overeating later. Stick to your regular eating schedule and choose healthy options throughout the day.
- **Stay Hydrated:** Drinking plenty of water can help curb cravings and keep you feeling full. Aim for eight glasses of water per day.
- **Communicate:** Communicate your goals to friends and family. Let them know you're trying to make healthy choices and politely decline unwanted pressure to indulge.
- **Focus on the Fun:** Holidays and vacations are about spending time with loved ones and creating memories. Focus on enjoying the festivities in healthy ways, like going for walks or participating in active games.
- **Prioritize Sleep:** Even during busy times, prioritize getting enough sleep. Adequate sleep is essential for stress management and regulating hormones that impact weight management.
- **Manage Stress:** Develop healthy coping mechanisms to manage stress effectively. Techniques like yoga, meditation, deep breathing, or spending time in nature can be helpful.

- **Self-Compassion:** Be kind to yourself! Don't get discouraged if you experience a setback. Acknowledge the challenge, learn from it, and recommit to your goals.
- **Celebrate Non-Scale Victories:** Did you resist temptation at a party? Did you manage to squeeze in a short workout during a busy week? Celebrate these non-scale victories! They are a testament to your progress and commitment.
- **Get Back on Track Quickly:** If you do overindulge, don't let it derail you. Get back on track with your healthy habits at your next meal or workout. Remember, one setback doesn't define your journey.
- **Enjoy the Journey:** Focus on making healthy choices that nourish your body and make you feel good. Find ways to make healthy eating and exercise enjoyable habits you can integrate into your lifestyle for the long term.

Remember, life will always throw curveballs. But by planning ahead, adopting a flexible mindset, and prioritizing your well-being, you can navigate these challenges and stay on track towards your weight loss and overall health goals. Embrace the journey, celebrate your victories, and live a happy, healthy life!

www.ingramcontent.com/pod-product-compliance
Lightning Source LLC
Chambersburg PA
CBHW031327250726
48656CB00005B/2001